GW01117102

DASH DIET COOKBOOK

2021

LOW SODIUM EASY RECIPES TO SPEED WEIGHT LOSS AND LOWER BLOOD PRESSURE

JENNA SCHULTZ

Table of Contents

Mustard Greens Sauté 8

Bok Choy Mix 9

Green Beans and Eggplant Mix 10

Olives and Artichokes Mix 11

Turmeric Peppers Dip 12

Lentils Spread 13

Roasted Walnuts 14

Cranberry Squares 15

Cauliflower Bars 16

Almonds and Seeds Bowls 17

Potato Chips 18

Kale Dip 19

Beets Chips 20

Zucchini Dip 21

Seeds and Apple Mix 22

Pumpkin Spread 23

Spinach Spread 24

Olives and Cilantro Salsa 25

Chives and Beets Dip 26

Cucumber Salsa 27

Chickpeas Dip 28

Olives Dip 29

Coconut Onions Dip 30

Pine Nuts and Coconut Dip 31

Arugula and Cucumbers Salsa	32
Cheese Dip	33
Paprika Yogurt Dip	34
Cauliflower Salsa	35
Shrimp Spread	36
Peach Salsa	37
Carrot Chips	38
Asparagus Bites	39
Baked Figs Bowls	40
Cabbage and Shrimp Salsa	41
Avocado Wedges	42
Lemon Dip	43
Sweet Potato Dip	44
Beans Salsa	45
Green Beans Salsa	46
Carrot Spread	47
Tomato Dip	48
Salmon Bowls	49
Tomato and Corn Salsa	50
Baked Mushrooms	51
Beans Spread	52
Coriander Fennel Salsa	53
Brussels Sprouts Bites	54
Balsamic Walnuts Bites	55
Radish Chips	56
Leeks and Shrimp Salad	57
Leeks Dip	58

Bell Peppers Slaw	59
Avocado Spread	60
Corn Dip	61
Beans Bars	62
Pumpkin Seeds and Apple Chips Mix	63
Tomatoes and Yogurt Dip	64
Cayenne Beet Bowls	65
Walnuts and Pecans Bowls	66
Parsley Salmon Muffins	67
Squash Balls	68
Cheesy Pearl Onion Bowls	69
Broccoli Bars	70
Pineapple and Tomato Salsa	71
Turkey and Artichokes Mix	72
Oregano Turkey Mix	73
Orange Chicken	74
Garlic Turkey and Mushrooms	75
Chicken and Olives Pan	76
Balsamic Turkey and Peach Mix	77
Coconut Chicken and Spinach	78
Chicken and Asparagus Mix	79
Turkey and Creamy Broccoli	80
Chicken and Dill Green Beans Mix	81
Chicken and Chili Zucchini	82
Avocado and Chicken Mix	84
Turkey and Bok Choy	85
Chicken with Red Onion Mix	86

Hot Turkey and Rice	87
Lemony Leek and Chicken	89
Turkey with Savoy Cabbage Mix	90
Chicken with Paprika Scallions	91
Chicken and Mustard Sauce	92
Chicken and Celery Mix	93
Lime Turkey with Baby Potatoes	94
Chicken with Mustard Greens	96
Baked Chicken and Apples	97
Chipotle Chicken	99
Herbed Turkey	101
Chicken and Ginger Sauce	102
Chicken and Corn	103
Curry Turkey and Quinoa	104
Turkey and Cumin Parsnips	105
Turkey and Cilantro Chickpeas	106
Turkey with Beans and Olives	108
Chicken and Tomato Quinoa	109
Allspice Chicken Wings	110
Chicken and Snow Peas	111

Mustard Greens Sauté

Preparation time: 10 minutes
Cooking time: 12 minutes
Servings: 4

Ingredients:
- 6 cups mustard greens
- 2 tablespoons olive oil
- 2 spring onions, chopped
- ½ cup coconut cream
- 2 tablespoons sweet paprika
- Black pepper to the taste

Directions:
1. Heat up a pan with the oil over medium-high heat, add the onions, paprika and black pepper, stir and sauté for 3 minutes.
2. Add the mustard greens and the other ingredients, toss, cook for 9 minutes more, divide between plates and serve as a side dish.

Nutrition: calories 163, fat 14.8, fiber 4.9, carbs 8.3, protein 3.6

Bok Choy Mix

Preparation time: 10 minutes
Cooking time: 12 minutes
Servings: 4

Ingredients:
- 1 tablespoon avocado oil
- 1 tablespoon balsamic vinegar
- 1 yellow onion, chopped
- 1 pound bok choy, torn
- 1 teaspoon cumin, ground
- 1 tablespoon coconut aminos
- ¼ cup low-sodium veggie stock
- Black pepper to the taste

Directions:
1. Heat up a pan with the oil over medium-high heat, add the onion, cumin and black pepper, stir and cook for 3 minutes.
2. Add the bok choy and the other ingredients, toss, cook for 8-9 minutes more, divide between plates and serve as a side dish.

Nutrition: calories 38, fat 0.8, fiber 2, carbs 6.5, protein 2.2

Green Beans and Eggplant Mix

Preparation time: 4 minutes
Cooking time: 40 minutes
Servings: 4

Ingredients:
- 1 pound green beans, trimmed and halved
- 1 small eggplant, cut into large chunks
- 1 yellow onion, chopped
- 2 tablespoons olive oil
- 2 tablespoons lime juice
- 1 teaspoon smoked paprika
- ¼ cup low-sodium veggie stock
- Black pepper to the taste
- ½ teaspoon oregano, dried

Directions:
1. In a roasting pan, combine the green beans with the eggplant and the other ingredients, toss, introduce in the oven, bake at 390 degrees F for 40 minutes, divide between plates and serve as a side dish.

Nutrition: calories 141, fat 7.5, fiber 8.9, carbs 19, protein 3.7

Olives and Artichokes Mix

Preparation time: 5 minutes
Cooing time: 0 minutes
Servings: 4

Ingredients:
- 10 ounces canned artichoke hearts, no-salt-added, drained and halved
- 1 cup black olives, pitted and sliced
- 1 tablespoon capers, drained
- 1 cup green olives, pitted and sliced
- 1 tablespoon parsley, chopped
- Black pepper to the taste
- 2 tablespoons olive oil
- 2 tablespoons red wine vinegar
- 1 tablespoon chives, chopped

Directions:
1. In a salad bowl, combine the artichokes with the olives and the other ingredients, toss and serve as a side dish.

Nutrition: calories 138, fat 11, fiber 5.1, carbs 10, protein 2.7

Turmeric Peppers Dip

Preparation time: 4 minutes
Cooking time: 0 minutes
Servings: 4

Ingredients:
- 1 teaspoon turmeric powder
- 1 cup coconut cream
- 14 ounces red peppers, no-salt-added, chopped
- Juice of ½ lemon
- 1 tablespoon chives, chopped

Directions:
1. In your blender, combine the peppers with the turmeric and the other ingredients except the chives, pulse well, divide into bowls and serve as a snack with the chives sprinkled on top.

Nutrition: calories 183, fat 14.9, fiber 3. carbs 12.7, protein 3.4

Lentils Spread

Preparation time: 5 minutes
Cooking time: 0 minutes
Servings: 4

Ingredients:
- 14 ounces canned lentils, drained, no-salt-added, rinsed
- Juice of 1 lemon
- 2 garlic cloves, minced
- 2 tablespoons olive oil
- ½ cup cilantro, chopped

Directions:
1. In a blender, combine the lentils with the oil and the other ingredients, pulse well, divide into bowls and serve as a party spread.

Nutrition: calories 416, fat 8.2, fiber 30.4, carbs 60.4, protein 25.8

Roasted Walnuts

Preparation time: 5 minutes
Cooking time: 15 minutes
Servings: 8

Ingredients:
- ½ teaspoon smoked paprika
- ½ teaspoon chili powder
- ½ teaspoon garlic powder
- 1 tablespoon avocado oil
- A pinch of cayenne pepper
- 14 ounces walnuts

Directions:
1. Spread the walnuts on a lined baking sheet, add the paprika and the other ingredients, toss and bake at 410 degrees F for 15 minutes.
2. Divide into bowls and serve as a snack.

Nutrition: calories 311, fat 29.6, fiber 3.6, carbs 5.3, protein 12

Cranberry Squares

Preparation time: 3 hours and 5 minutes

Cooking time: 0 minutes
Servings: 4

Ingredients:
- 2 ounces coconut cream
- 2 tablespoons rolled oats
- 2 tablespoons coconut, shredded
- 1 cup cranberries

Directions:
1. In a blender, combine the oats with the cranberries and the other ingredients, pulse well and spread into a square pan.

Cut into squares and keep them in the fridge for 3 hours before serving.

Nutrition: calories 66, fat 4.4, fiber 1.8, carbs 5.4, protein 0.8

Cauliflower Bars

Preparation time: 10 minutes
Cooking time: 30 minutes
Servings: 8

Ingredients:
- 2 cups whole wheat flour
- 2 teaspoons baking powder
- A pinch of black pepper
- 2 eggs, whisked
- 1 cup almond milk
- 1 cup cauliflower florets, chopped
- ½ cup low-fat cheddar, shredded

Directions:
1. In a bowl, combine the flour with the cauliflower and the other ingredients and stir well.
2. Spread into a baking tray, introduce in the oven, bake at 400 degrees F for 30 minutes, cut into bars and serve as a snack.

Nutrition: calories 430, fat 18.1, fiber 3.7, carbs 54, protein 14.5

Almonds and Seeds Bowls

Preparation time: 5 minutes
Cooking time: 10 minutes
Servings: 4

Ingredients:
- 2 cups almonds
- ¼ cup coconut, shredded
- 1 mango, peeled and cubed
- 1 cup sunflower seeds
- Cooking spray

Directions:
1. Spread the almonds, coconut, mango and sunflower seeds on a baking tray, grease with the cooking spray, toss and bake at 400 degrees F for 10 minutes.
2. Divide into bowls and serve as a snack.

Nutrition: calories 411, fat 31.8, fiber 8.7, carbs 25.8, protein 13.3

Potato Chips

Preparation time: 10 minutes
Cooking time: 20 minutes
Servings: 4

Ingredients:
- 4 gold potatoes, peeled and thinly sliced
- 2 tablespoons olive oil
- 1 tablespoon chili powder
- 1 teaspoon sweet paprika
- 1 tablespoon chives, chopped

Directions:
1. Spread the chips on a lined baking sheet, add the oil and the other ingredients, toss, introduce in the oven and bake at 390 degrees F for 20 minutes.
2. Divide into bowls and serve.

Nutrition: calories 118, fat 7.4, fiber 2.9, carbs 13.4, protein 1.3

Kale Dip

Preparation time: 10 minutes
Cooking time: 20 minutes
Servings: 4

Ingredients:
- 1 bunch kale leaves
- 1 cup coconut cream
- 1 shallot, chopped
- 1 tablespoon olive oil
- 1 teaspoon chili powder
- A pinch of black pepper

Directions:
1. Heat up a pan with the oil over medium heat, add the shallots, stir and sauté for 4 minutes.
2. Add the kale and the other ingredients, bring to a simmer and cook over medium heat for 16 minutes.
3. Blend using an immersion blender, divide into bowls and serve as a snack.

Nutrition: calories 188, fat 17.9, fiber 2.1, carbs 7.6, protein 2.5

Beets Chips

Preparation time: 10 minutes
Cooking time: 35 minutes
Servings: 4

Ingredients:
- 2 beets, peeled and thinly sliced
- 1 tablespoon avocado oil
- 1 teaspoon cumin, ground
- 1 teaspoon fennel seeds, crushed
- 2 teaspoons garlic, minced

Directions:
1. Spread the beet chips on a lined baking sheet, add the oil and the other ingredients, toss, introduce in the oven and bake at 400 degrees F for 35 minutes.
2. Divide into bowls and serve as a snack.

Nutrition: calories 32, fat 0.7, fiber 1.4, carbs 6.1, protein 1.1

Zucchini Dip

Preparation time: 5 minutes
Cooking time: 10 minutes
Servings: 4

Ingredients:
- ½ cup nonfat yogurt
- 2 zucchinis, chopped
- 1 tablespoon olive oil
- 2 spring onions, chopped
- ¼ cup low-sodium veggie stock
- 2 garlic cloves, minced
- 1 tablespoon dill, chopped
- A pinch of nutmeg, ground

Directions:
1. Heat up a pan with the oil over medium heat, add the onions and garlic, stir and sauté for 3 minutes.
2. Add the zucchinis and the other ingredients except the yogurt, toss, cook for 7 minutes more and take off the heat.
3. Add the yogurt, blend using an immersion blender, divide into bowls and serve.

Nutrition: calories 76, fat 4.1, fiber 1.5, carbs 7.2, protein 3.4

Seeds and Apple Mix

Preparation time: 10 minutes
Cooking time: 20 minutes
Servings: 4

Ingredients:
- 2 tablespoons olive oil
- 1 teaspoon smoked paprika
- 1 cup sunflower seeds
- 1 cup chia seeds
- 2 apples, cored and cut into wedges
- ½ teaspoon cumin, ground
- A pinch of cayenne pepper

Directions:
1. In a bowl, combine the seeds with the apples and the other ingredients, toss, spread on a lined baking sheet, introduce in the oven and bake at 350 degrees F for 20 minutes.
2. Divide into bowls and serve as a snack.

Nutrition: calories 222, fat 15.4, fiber 6.4, carbs 21.1, protein 4

Pumpkin Spread

Preparation time: 5 minutes
Cooking time: 0 minutes
Servings: 4

Ingredients:
- 2 cups pumpkin flesh
- ½ cup pumpkin seeds
- 1 tablespoon lemon juice
- 1 tablespoon sesame seed paste
- 1 tablespoon olive oil

Directions:
1. In a blender, combine the pumpkin with the seeds and the other ingredients, pulse well, divide into bowls and serve a party spread.

Nutrition: calories 162, fat 12.7, fiber 2.3, carbs 9.7, protein 5.5

Spinach Spread

Preparation time: 10 minutes
Cooking time: 20 minutes
Servings: 4

Ingredients:
- 1 pound spinach, chopped
- 1 cup coconut cream
- 1 cup low-fat mozzarella, shredded
- A pinch of black pepper
- 1 tablespoon dill, chopped

Directions:
1. In a baking pan, combine the spinach with the cream and the other ingredients, stir well, introduce in the oven and bake at 400 degrees F for 20 minutes.
2. Divide into bowls and serve.

Nutrition: calories 186, fat 14.8, fiber 4.4, carbs 8.4, protein 8.8

Olives and Cilantro Salsa

Preparation time: 5 minutes
Cooking time: 0 minutes
Servings: 4

Ingredients:
- 1 red onion, chopped
- 1 cup black olives, pitted and halved
- 1 cucumber, cubed
- ¼ cup cilantro, chopped
- A pinch of black pepper
- 2 tablespoons lime juice

Directions:
1. In a bowl, combine the olives with the cucumber and the rest of the ingredients, toss and serve cold as a snack.

Nutrition: calories 64, fat 3.7, fiber 2.1, carbs 8.4, protein 1.1

Chives and Beets Dip

Preparation time: 5 minutes
Cooking time: 25 minutes
Servings: 4

Ingredients:
- 2 tablespoons olive oil
- 1 red onion, chopped
- 2 tablespoons chives, chopped
- A pinch of black pepper
- 1 beet, peeled and chopped
- 8 ounces low-fat cream cheese
- 1 cup coconut cream

Directions:
1. Heat up a pan with the oil over medium heat, add the onion and sauté for 5 minutes.
2. Add the rest of the ingredients, and cook everything for 20 minutes more stirring often.
3. Transfer the mix to a blender, pulse well, divide into bowls and serve.

Nutrition: calories 418, fat 41.2, fiber 2.5, carbs 10, protein 6.4

Cucumber Salsa

Preparation time: 5 minutes
Cooking time: 0 minutes
Servings: 4

Ingredients:
- 1 pound cucumbers cubed
- 1 avocado, peeled, pitted and cubed
- 1 tablespoon capers, drained
- 1 tablespoon chives, chopped
- 1 small red onion, cubed
- 1 tablespoon olive oil
- 1 tablespoon balsamic vinegar

Directions:
1. In a bowl, combine the cucumbers with the avocado and the other ingredients, toss, divide into small cups and serve.

Nutrition: calories 132, fat 4.4, fiber 4, carbs 11.6, protein 4.5

Chickpeas Dip

Preparation time: 5 minutes
Cooking time: 0 minutes
Servings: 4

Ingredients:
- 1 tablespoon olive oil
- 1 tablespoon lemon juice
- 1 tablespoon sesame seeds paste
- 2 tablespoons chives, chopped
- 2 spring onions, chopped
- 2 cups canned chickpeas, no-salt-added, drained and rinsed

Directions:
1. In your blender, combine the chickpeas with the oil and the other ingredients except the chives, pulse well, divide into bowls, sprinkle the chives on top and serve.

Nutrition: calories 280, fat 13.3, fiber 5.5, carbs 14.8, protein 6.2

Olives Dip

Preparation time: 4 minutes
Cooking time: 0 minutes
Servings: 4

Ingredients:
- 2 cups black olives, pitted and chopped
- 1 cup mint, chopped
- 2 tablespoons avocado oil
- ½ cup coconut cream
- ¼ cup lime juice
- A pinch of black pepper

Directions:
1. In your blender, combine the olives with the mint and the other ingredients, pulse well, divide into bowls and serve.

Nutrition: calories 287, fat 13.3, fiber 4.7, carbs 17.4, protein 2.4

Coconut Onions Dip

Preparation time: 5 minutes
Cooking time: 0 minutes
Servings: 4

Ingredients:
- 4 spring onions, chopped
- 1 shallot, minced
- 1 tablespoon lime juice
- A pinch of black pepper
- 2 ounces low-fat mozzarella cheese, shredded
- 1 cup coconut cream
- 1 tablespoon parsley, chopped

Directions:
1. In a blender, combine the spring onions with the shallot and the other ingredients, pulse well, divide into bowls and serve as a party dip.

Nutrition: calories 271, fat 15.3, fiber 5, carbs 15.9, protein 6.9

Pine Nuts and Coconut Dip

Preparation time: 5 minutes
Cooking time: 0 minutes
Servings: 4

Ingredients:
- 8 ounces coconut cream
- 1 tablespoon pine nuts, chopped
- 2 tablespoons parsley, chopped
- A pinch of black pepper

Directions:
1. In a bowl, combine the cream with the pine nuts and the rest of the ingredients, whisk well, divide into bowls and serve.

Nutrition: calories 281, fat 13, fiber 4.8, carbs 16, protein 3.56

Arugula and Cucumbers Salsa

Preparation time: 5 minutes
Cooking time: 0 minutes
Servings: 4

Ingredients:
- 4 scallions, chopped
- 2 tomatoes, cubed
- 4 cucumbers, cubed
- 1 tablespoon balsamic vinegar
- 1 cup baby arugula leaves
- 2 tablespoons lemon juice
- 2 tablespoons olive oil
- A pinch of black pepper

Directions:
1. In a bowl, combine the scallions with the tomatoes and the other ingredients, toss, divide into small bowls and serve as a snack.

Nutrition: calories 139, fat 3.8, fiber 4.5, carbs 14, protein 5.4

Cheese Dip

Preparation time: 5 minutes
Cooking time: 0 minutes
Servings: 6

Ingredients:
- 1 tablespoon mint, chopped
- 1 tablespoon oregano, chopped
- 10 ounces non-fat cream cheese
- ½ cup ginger, sliced
- 2 tablespoons coconut aminos

Directions:
1. In your blender, combine the cream cheese with the ginger and the other ingredients, pulse well, divide into small cups and serve.

Nutrition: calories 388, fat 15.4, fiber 6, carbs 14.3, protein 6

Paprika Yogurt Dip

Preparation time: 5 minutes
Cooking time: 0 minutes
Servings: 4

Ingredients:
- 3 cups non-fat yogurt
- 2 spring onions, chopped
- 1 teaspoon sweet paprika
- ¼ cup almonds, chopped
- ¼ cup dill, chopped

Directions:
1. In a bowl, combine the yogurt with the onions and the other ingredients, whisk, divide into bowls and serve.

Nutrition: calories 181, fat 12.2, fiber 6, carbs 14,1, protein 7

Cauliflower Salsa

Preparation time: 5 minutes
Cooking time: 0 minutes
Servings: 4

Ingredients:
- 1 pound cauliflower florets, blanched
- 1 cup kalamata olives, pitted and halved
- 1 cup cherry tomatoes, halved
- 1 tablespoon olive oil
- 1 tablespoon lime juice
- A pinch of black pepper

Directions:
1. In a bowl, combine the cauliflower with the olives and the other ingredients, toss and serve.

Nutrition: calories 139, fat 4, fiber 3.6, carbs 5.5, protein 3.4

Shrimp Spread

Preparation time: 5 minutes
Cooking time: 0 minutes
Servings: 4

Ingredients:
- 8 ounces coconut cream
- 1 pound shrimp, cooked, peeled, deveined and chopped
- 2 tablespoons dill, chopped
- 2 spring onions, chopped
- 1 tablespoon cilantro, chopped
- A pinch of black pepper

Directions:
1. In a bowl, combine the shrimp with the cream and the other ingredients, whisk and serve as a party spread.

Nutrition: calories 362, fat 14.3, fiber 6, carbs 14.6, protein 5.9

Peach Salsa

Preparation time: 4 minutes
Cooking time: 0 minutes
Servings: 4

Ingredients:
- 4 peaches, stones removed and cubed
- 1 cup kalamata olives, pitted and halved
- 1 avocado, pitted, peeled and cubed
- 1 cup cherry tomatoes, halved
- 1 tablespoon olive oil
- 1 tablespoon lime juice
- 1 tablespoon cilantro, chopped

Directions:
1. In a bowl, combine the peaches with the olives and the other ingredients, toss well and serve cold.

Nutrition: calories 200, fat 7.5, fiber 5, carbs 13.3, protein 4.9

Carrot Chips

Preparation time: 10 minutes
Cooking time: 20 minutes
Servings: 4

Ingredients:
- 4 carrots, thinly sliced
- 2 tablespoons olive oil
- A pinch of black pepper
- 1 teaspoon sweet paprika
- ½ teaspoon turmeric powder
- A pinch of red pepper flakes

Directions:
1. In a bowl, combine the carrot chips with the oil and the other ingredients and toss.
2. Spread the chips on a lined baking sheet, bake at 400 degrees F for 25 minutes, divide into bowls and serve as a snack.

Nutrition: calories 180, fat 3, fiber 3.3, carbs 5.8, protein 1.3

Asparagus Bites

Preparation time: 4 minutes
Cooking time: 20 minutes
Servings: 4

Ingredients:
- 2 tablespoons coconut oil, melted
- 1 pound asparagus, trimmed and halved
- 1 teaspoon garlic powder
- 1 teaspoon rosemary, dried
- 1 teaspoon chili powder

Directions:
1. In a bowl, mix the asparagus with the oil and the other ingredients, toss, spread on a lined baking sheet and bake at 400 degrees F for 20 minutes.
2. Divide into bowls and serve cold as a snack.

Nutrition: calories 170, fat 4.3, fiber 4, carbs 7, protein 4.5

Baked Figs Bowls

Preparation time: 4 minutes
Cooking time: 12 minutes
Servings: 4

Ingredients:
- 8 figs, halved
- 1 tablespoon avocado oil
- 1 teaspoon nutmeg, ground

Directions:
1. In a roasting pan combine the figs with the oil and the nutmeg, toss, and bake at 400 degrees F for 12 minutes.
2. Divide the figs into small bowls and serve as a snack.

Nutrition: calories 180, fat 4.3, fiber 2, carbs 2, protein 3.2

Cabbage and Shrimp Salsa

Preparation time: 5 minutes
Cooking time: 6 minutes
Servings: 4

Ingredients:
- 2 cups red cabbage, shredded
- 1 pound shrimp, peeled and deveined
- 1 tablespoon olive oil
- A pinch of black pepper
- 2 spring onions, chopped
- 1 cup tomatoes, cubed
- ½ teaspoon garlic powder

Directions:
1. Heat up a pan with the oil over medium heat, add the shrimp, toss and cook for 3 minutes on each side.
2. In a bowl, combine the cabbage with the shrimp and the other ingredients, toss, divide into small bowls and serve.

Nutrition: calories 225, fat 9.7, fiber 5.1, carbs 11.4, protein 4.5

Avocado Wedges

Preparation time: 5 minutes
Cooking time: 10 minutes
Servings: 4

Ingredients:
- 2 avocados, peeled, pitted and cut into wedges
- 1 tablespoon avocado oil
- 1 tablespoon lime juice
- 1 teaspoon coriander, ground

Directions:
1. Spread the avocado wedges on a lined baking sheet, add the oil and the other ingredients, toss, and bake at 300 degrees F for 10 minutes.
2. Divide into cups and serve as a snack.

Nutrition: calories 212, fat 20.1, fiber 6.9, carbs 9.8, protein 2

Lemon Dip

Preparation time: 4 minutes
Cooking time: 0 minutes
Servings: 4

Ingredients:
- 1 cup low-fat cream cheese
- Black pepper to the taste
- ½ cup lemon juice
- 1 tablespoon cilantro, chopped
- 3 garlic cloves, chopped

Directions:
1. In your food processor, mix the cream cheese with the lemon juice and the other ingredients, pulse well, divide into bowls and serve.

Nutrition: calories 213, fat 20.5, fiber 0.2, carbs 2.8, protein 4.8

Sweet Potato Dip

Preparation time: 10 minutes
Cooking time: 40 minutes
Servings: 4

Ingredients:
- 1 cup sweet potatoes, peeled and cubed
- 1 tablespoon low-sodium veggie stock
- Cooking spray
- 2 tablespoons coconut cream
- 2 teaspoons rosemary, dried
- Black pepper to the taste

Directions:
1. In a baking pan, combine the potatoes with the stock and the other ingredients, stir, bake at 365 degrees F for 40 minutes, transfer to your blender, pulse well, divide into small bowls and serve

Nutrition: calories 65, fat 2.1, fiber 2, carbs 11.3, protein 0.8

Beans Salsa

Preparation time: 5 minutes
Cooking time: 0 minutes
Servings: 4

Ingredients:
- 1 cup canned black beans, no-salt-added, drained
- 1 cup canned red kidney beans, no-salt-added, drained
- 1 teaspoon balsamic vinegar
- 1 cup cherry tomatoes, cubed
- 1 tablespoon olive oil
- 2 shallots, chopped

Directions:
1. In a bowl, combine the beans with the vinegar and the other ingredients, toss and serve as a party snack.

Nutrition: calories 362, fat 4.8, fiber 14.9, carbs 61, protein 21.4

Green Beans Salsa

Preparation time: 10 minutes
Cooking time: 10 minutes
Servings: 4

Ingredients:
- 1 pound green beans, trimmed and halved
- 1 tablespoon olive oil
- 2 teaspoons capers, drained
- 6 ounces green olives, pitted and sliced
- 4 garlic cloves, minced
- 1 tablespoon lime juice
- 1 tablespoon oregano, chopped
- Black pepper to the taste

Directions:
1. Heat up a pan with the oil over medium-high heat, add the garlic and the green beans, toss and cook for 3 minutes.
2. Add the rest of the ingredients, toss, cook for another 7 minutes, divide into small cups and serve cold.

Nutrition: calories 111, fat 6.7, fiber 5.6, carbs 13.2, protein 2.9

Carrot Spread

Preparation time: 10 minutes
Cooking time: 30 minutes
Servings: 4

Ingredients:
- 1 pound carrots, peeled and chopped
- ½ cup walnuts, chopped
- 2 cups low-sodium veggie stock
- 1 cup coconut cream
- 1 tablespoon rosemary, chopped
- 1 teaspoon garlic powder
- ¼ teaspoon smoked paprika

Directions:
1. In a small pot, mix the carrots with the stock, walnuts and the other ingredients except the cream and the rosemary, stir, bring to a boil over medium heat, cook for 30 minutes, drain and transfer to a blender.
2. Add the cream, blend the mix well, divide into bowls, sprinkle the rosemary on top and serve.

Nutrition: calories 201, fat 8.7, fiber 3.4, carbs 7.8, protein 7.7

Tomato Dip

Preparation time: 10 minutes
Cooking time: 10 minutes
Servings: 4

Ingredients:
- 1 pound tomatoes, peeled and chopped
- ½ cup garlic, minced
- 2 tablespoons olive oil
- A pinch of black pepper
- 2 shallots, chopped
- 1 teaspoon thyme, dried

Directions:
1. Heat up a pan with the oil over medium-high heat, add the garlic and the shallots, stir and sauté for 2 minutes.
2. Add the tomatoes and the other ingredients, cook for 8 minutes more and transfer to a blender.
3. Pulse well, divide into small cups and serve as a snack.

Nutrition: calories 232, fat 11.3, fiber 3.9, carbs 7.9, protein 4.5

Salmon Bowls

Preparation time: 10 minutes
Cooking time: 0 minutes
Servings: 6

Ingredients:
- 1 tablespoon avocado oil
- 1 tablespoon balsamic vinegar
- ½ teaspoon oregano, dried
- 1 cup smoked salmon, no-salt-added, boneless, skinless and cubed
- 1 cup salsa
- 4 cups baby spinach

Directions:
1. In a bowl, combine the salmon with the salsa and the other ingredients, toss, divide into small cups and serve.

Nutrition: calories 281, fat 14.4, fiber 7.4, carbs 18.7, protein 7.4

Tomato and Corn Salsa

Preparation time: 4 minutes
Cooking time: 0 minutes
Servings: 4

Ingredients:
- 3 cups corn
- 2 cups tomatoes, cubed
- 2 green onions, chopped
- 2 tablespoons olive oil
- 1 red chili pepper, chopped
- ½ tablespoon chives, chopped

Directions:
1. In a salad bowl, combine the tomatoes with the corn and the other ingredients, toss and serve cold as a snack.

Nutrition: calories 178, fat 8.6, fiber 4.5, carbs 25.9, protein 4.7

Baked Mushrooms

Preparation time: 10 minutes
Cooking time: 25 minutes
Servings: 4

Ingredients:
- 1 pound small mushroom caps
- 2 tablespoons olive oil
- 1 tablespoon chives, chopped
- 1 tablespoon rosemary, chopped
- Black pepper to the taste

Directions:
1. Put the mushrooms in a roasting pan, add the oil and the rest of the ingredients, toss, bake at 400 degrees F for 25 minutes, divide into bowls and serve as a snack.

Nutrition: calories 215, fat 12.3, fiber 6.7, carbs 15.3, protein 3.5

Beans Spread

Preparation time: 5 minutes
Cooking time: 0 minutes
Servings: 4

Ingredients:
- ½ cup coconut cream
- 1 tablespoon olive oil
- 2 cups canned black beans, no-salt-added, drained and rinsed
- 2 tablespoons green onions, chopped

Directions:
1. In a blender, combine the beans with the cream and the other ingredients, pulse well, divide into bowls and serve.

Nutrition: calories 311, fat 13.5, fiber 6, carbs 18.0, protein 8

Coriander Fennel Salsa

Preparation time: 5 minutes
Cooking time: 0 minutes
Servings: 4

Ingredients:
- 2 spring onion, chopped
- 2 fennel bulbs, shredded
- 1 green chili pepper, chopped
- 1 tomato, chopped
- 1 teaspoon turmeric powder
- 1 teaspoon lime juice
- 2 tablespoons coriander, chopped
- Black pepper to the taste

Directions:
1. In a salad bowl, mix the fennel with the onions and the other ingredients, toss, divide into cups and serve.

Nutrition: calories 310, fat 11.5, fiber 5.1, carbs 22.3, protein 6.5

Brussels Sprouts Bites

Preparation time: 10 minutes
Cooking time: 25 minutes
Servings: 4

Ingredients:
- 1 pound Brussels sprouts, trimmed and halved
- 2 tablespoons olive oil
- 1 tablespoon cumin, ground
- 1 cup dill, chopped
- 2 garlic cloves, minced

Directions:
1. In a roasting pan, combine the Brussels sprouts with the oil and the other ingredients, toss and bake at 390 degrees F for 25 minutes.
2. Divide the sprouts into bowls and serve as a snack.

Nutrition: calories 270, fat 10.3, fiber 5.2, carbs 11.1, protein 6

Balsamic Walnuts Bites

Preparation time: 10 minutes
Cooking time: 15 minutes
Servings: 4

Ingredients:
- 2 cups walnuts
- 3 tablespoons red vinegar
- A drizzle of olive oil
- A pinch of cayenne pepper
- A pinch of red pepper flakes
- Black pepper to the taste

Directions:
1. Spread the walnuts on a lined baking sheet, add the vinegar and the other ingredients, toss, and roast at 400 degrees F for 15 minutes.
2. Divide the walnuts into bowls and serve.

Nutrition: calories 280, fat 12.2, fiber 2, carbs 15.8, protein 6

Radish Chips

Preparation time: 10 minutes
Cooking time: 20 minutes
Servings: 4

Ingredients:
- 1 pound radishes, thinly sliced
- A pinch of turmeric powder
- Black pepper to the taste
- 2 tablespoons olive oil

Directions:
1. Spread the radish chips on a lined baking sheet, add the oil and the other ingredients, toss and bake at 400 degrees F for 20 minutes.
2. Divide the chips into bowls and serve.

Nutrition: calories 120, fat 8.3, fiber 1, carbs 3.8, protein 6

Leeks and Shrimp Salad

Preparation time: 4 minutes
Cooking time: 0 minutes
Servings: 4

Ingredients:
- 2 leeks, sliced
- 1 cup cilantro, chopped
- 1 pound shrimp, peeled, deveined and cooked
- Juice of 1 lime
- 1 tablespoon lime zest, grated
- 1 cup cherry tomatoes, halved
- 2 tablespoons olive oil
- Salt and black pepper to the taste

Directions:
1. In a salad bowl, mix the shrimp with the leeks and the other ingredients, toss, divide into small cups and serve.

Nutrition: calories 280, fat 9.1, fiber 5.2, carbs 12.6, protein 5

Leeks Dip

Preparation time: 5 minutes
Cooking time: 0 minutes
Servings: 4

Ingredients:
- 1 tablespoon lemon juice
- ½ cup low-fat cream cheese
- 2 tablespoons olive oil
- Black pepper to the taste
- 4 leeks, chopped
- 1 tablespoon cilantro, chopped

Directions:
1. In a blender, combine the cream cheese with the leeks and the other ingredients, pulse well, divide into bowls and serve as a party dip.

Nutrition: calories 300, fat 12.2, fiber 7.6, carbs 14.7, protein 5.6

Bell Peppers Slaw

Preparation time: 5 minutes
Cooking time: 0 minutes
Servings: 4

Ingredients:
- ½ pound red bell pepper, cut into thin strips
- 3 green onions, chopped
- 1 tablespoon olive oil
- 2 teaspoons ginger, grated
- ½ teaspoon rosemary, dried
- 3 tablespoons balsamic vinegar

Directions:
1. In a salad bowl, mix the bell peppers with the onions and the other ingredients, toss, divide into small cups and serve.

Nutrition: calories 160, fat 6, fiber 3, carbs 10.9, protein 5.2

Avocado Spread

Preparation time: 4 minutes
Cooking time: 0 minutes
Servings: 4

Ingredients:
- 2 tablespoons dill, chopped
- 1 shallot, chopped
- 2 garlic cloves, minced
- 2 avocados, peeled, pitted and chopped
- 1 cup coconut cream
- 2 tablespoons olive oil
- 2 tablespoons lime juice
- Black pepper to the taste

Directions:
1. In a blender, combine the avocados with the shallots, garlic and the other ingredients, pulse well, divide into small bowls and serve as a snack.

Nutrition: calories 300, fat 22.3, fiber 6.4, carbs 42, protein 8.9

Corn Dip

Preparation time: 30 minutes
Cooking time: 0 minutes
Servings: 4

Ingredients:
- A pinch of cayenne pepper
- A pinch of black pepper
- 2 cups corn
- 1 cup coconut cream
- 2 tablespoons lemon juice
- 2 tablespoon avocado oil

Directions:
1. In a blender, combine the corn with the cream and the other ingredients, pulse well, divide into bowls and serve as a party dip.

Nutrition: calories 215, fat 16.2, fiber 3.8, carbs 18.4, protein 4

Beans Bars

Preparation time: 2 hours
Cooking time: 0 minutes
Servings: 12

Ingredients:
- 1 cup canned black beans, no-salt-added, drained
- 1 cup coconut flakes, unsweetened
- 1 cup low-fat butter
- ½ cup chia seeds
- ½ cup coconut cream

Directions:
1. In a blender, combine the beans with the coconut flakes and the other ingredients, pulse well, spread this into a square pan, press, keep in the fridge for 2 hours, slice into medium bars and serve.

Nutrition: calories 141, fat 7, fiber 5, carbs 16.2, protein 5

Pumpkin Seeds and Apple Chips Mix

Preparation time: 10 minutes
Cooking time: 2 hours
Servings: 4

Ingredients:
- Cooking spray
- 2 teaspoons nutmeg, ground
- 1 cup pumpkin seeds
- 2 apples, cored and thinly sliced

Directions:
1. Arrange the pumpkin seeds and the apple chips on a lined baking sheet, sprinkle the nutmeg all over, grease them with the spray, introduce in the oven and bake at 300 degrees F for 2 hours.
2. Divide into bowls and serve as a snack.

Nutrition: calories 80, fat 0, fiber 3, carbs 7, protein 4

Tomatoes and Yogurt Dip

Preparation time: 5 minutes
Cooking time: 0 minutes
Servings: 4

Ingredients:
- 2 cups fat-free Greek yogurt
- 1 tablespoon parsley, chopped
- ¼ cup canned tomatoes, no-salt-added, chopped
- 2 tablespoons chives, chopped
- Black pepper to the taste

Directions:
1. In a bowl, mix the yogurt with the parsley and the other ingredients, whisk well, divide into small bowls and serve as a party dip.

Nutrition: calories 78, fat 0, fiber 0.2, carbs 10.6, protein 8.2

Cayenne Beet Bowls

Preparation time: 10 minutes
Cooking time: 35 minutes
Servings: 2

Ingredients:
- 1 teaspoon cayenne pepper
- 2 beets, peeled and cubed
- 1 teaspoon rosemary, dried
- 1 tablespoon olive oil
- 2 teaspoons lime juice

Directions:
1. In a roasting pan, combine the beet bites with the cayenne and the other ingredients, toss, introduce in the oven, roast at 355 degrees F for 35 minutes, divide into small bowls and serve as a snack.

Nutrition: calories 170, fat 12.2, fiber 7, carbs 15.1, protein 6

Walnuts and Pecans Bowls

Preparation time: 10 minutes
Cooking time: 10 minutes
Servings: 4

Ingredients:
- 2 cup walnuts
- 1 cup pecans, chopped
- 1 teaspoon avocado oil
- ½ teaspoon sweet paprika

Directions:
1. Spread the grapes and pecans on a lined baking sheet, add the oil and the paprika, toss, and bake at 400 degrees F for 10 minutes.
2. Divide into bowls and serve as a snack.

Nutrition: calories 220, fat 12.4, fiber 3, carbs 12.9, protein 5.6

Parsley Salmon Muffins

Preparation time: 10 minutes
Cooking time: 25 minutes
Servings: 4

Ingredients:
- 1 cup low-fat mozzarella cheese, shredded
- 8 ounces smoked salmon, skinless, boneless, and chopped
- 1 cup almond flour
- 1 egg, whisked
- 1 teaspoon parsley, dried
- 1 garlic clove, minced
- Black pepper to the taste
- Cooking spray

Directions:
1. In a bowl, combine the salmon with the mozzarella and the other ingredients except the cooking spray and stir well.
2. Divide this mix into a muffin tray greased with the cooking spray, bake in the oven at 375 degrees F for 25 minutes and serve as a snack.

Nutrition: calories 273, fat 17, fiber 3.5, carbs 6.9, protein 21.8

Squash Balls

Preparation time: 10 minutes
Cooking time: 20 minutes
Servings: 8

Ingredients:
- A drizzle of olive oil
- 1 big butternut squash, peeled and minced
- 2 tablespoons cilantro, chopped
- 2 eggs, whisked
- ½ cup whole wheat flour
- Black pepper to the taste
- 2 shallots, chopped
- 2 garlic cloves, minced

Directions:
1. In a bowl, mix the squash with the cilantro and the other ingredients except the oil, stir well and shape medium balls out of this mix.
2. Arrange them on a lined baking sheet, grease them with the oil, bake at 400 degrees F for 10 minutes on each side, divide into bowls and serve.

Nutrition: calories 78, fat 3, fiber 0.9, carbs 10.8, protein 2.7

Cheesy Pearl Onion Bowls

Preparation time: 10 minutes
Cooking time: 30 minutes
Servings: 8

Ingredients:
- 20 white pearl onions, peeled
- 3 tablespoons parsley, chopped
- 1 tablespoon chives, chopped
- Black pepper to the taste
- 1 cup low-fat mozzarella, grated
- 1 tablespoon olive oil

Directions:
1. Spread the pearl onions on a lined baking sheet, add the oil, parsley, chives and the black pepper and toss.
2. Sprinkle the mozzarella on top, bake at 390 degrees F for 30 minutes, divide into bowls and serve cold as a snack.

Nutrition: calories 136, fat 2.7, fiber 6, carbs 25.9, protein 4.1

Broccoli Bars

Preparation time: 10 minutes
Cooking time: 25 minutes
Servings: 8

Ingredients:
- 1 pound broccoli florets, chopped
- ½ cup low-fat mozzarella cheese, shredded
- 2 eggs, whisked
- 1 teaspoon oregano, dried
- 1 teaspoon basil, dried
- Black pepper to the taste

Directions:
1. In a bowl, mix the broccoli with the cheese and the other ingredients, stir well, spread into a rectangle pan and press well on the bottom.
2. Introduce in the oven at 380 degrees F, bake for 25 minutes, cut into bars and serve cold.

Nutrition: calories 46, fat 1.3, fiber 1.8, carbs 4.2, protein 5

Pineapple and Tomato Salsa

Preparation time: 10 minutes
Cooking time: 40 minutes
Servings: 4

Ingredients:
- 20 ounces canned pineapple, drained and cubed
- 1 cup sun-dried tomatoes, cubed
- 1 tablespoon basil, chopped
- 1 tablespoon avocado oil
- 1 teaspoon lime juice
- 1 cup black olives, pitted and sliced
- Black pepper to the taste

Directions:
1. In a bowl, combine the pineapple cubes with the tomatoes and the other ingredients, toss, divide into smaller cups and serve as a snack.

Nutrition: calories 125, fat 4.3, fiber 3.8, carbs 23.6, protein 1.5

Turkey and Artichokes Mix

Preparation time: 5 minutes
Cooking time: 25 minutes
Servings: 4

Ingredients:
- 2 tablespoons olive oil
- 1 turkey breast, skinless, boneless and sliced
- A pinch of black pepper
- 1 tablespoon basil, chopped
- 3 garlic cloves, minced
- 14 ounces canned artichokes, no-salt-added, chopped
- 1 cup coconut cream
- ¾ cup low-fat mozzarella, shredded

Directions:
1. Heat up a pan with the oil over medium-high heat, add the meat, garlic and the black pepper, toss and cook for 5 minutes.
2. Add the rest of the ingredients except the cheese, toss and cook over medium heat for 15 minutes.
3. Sprinkle the cheese, cook everything for 5 minutes more, divide between plates and serve.

Nutrition: calories 300, fat 22.2, fiber 7.2, carbs 16.5, protein 13.6

Oregano Turkey Mix

Preparation time: 10 minutes
Cooking time: 30 minutes
Servings: 4

Ingredients:
- 2 tablespoons avocado oil
- 1 red onion, chopped
- 2 garlic cloves, minced
- A pinch of black pepper
- 1 tablespoon oregano, chopped
- 1 big turkey breast, skinless, boneless and cubed
- 1 and ½ cups low-sodium beef stock
- 1 tablespoon chives, chopped

Directions:
1. Heat up a pan with the oil over medium heat, add the onion, stir and sauté for 3 minutes.
2. Add the garlic and the meat, toss and cook for 3 minutes more.
3. Add the rest of the ingredients, toss, simmer everything over medium heat fro 25 minutes, divide between plates and serve.

Nutrition: calories 76, fat 2.1, fiber 1.7, carbs 6.4, protein 8.3

Orange Chicken

Preparation time: 10 minutes
Cooking time: 35 minutes
Servings: 4

Ingredients:
- 1 tablespoon avocado oil
- 1 pound chicken breast, skinless, boneless and halved
- 2 garlic cloves, minced
- 2 shallots, chopped
- ½ cup orange juice
- 1 tablespoon orange zest, grated
- 3 tablespoons balsamic vinegar
- 1 teaspoon rosemary, chopped

Directions:
1. Heat up a pan with the oil over medium-high heat, add the shallots and the garlic, toss and sauté for 2 minutes.
2. Add the meat, toss gently and cook for 3 minutes more.
3. Add the rest of the ingredients, toss, introduce the pan in the oven and bake at 340 degrees F for 30 minutes.
4. Divide between plates and serve.

Nutrition: calories 159, fat 3.4, fiber 0.5, carbs 5.4, protein 24.6

Garlic Turkey and Mushrooms

Preparation time: 10 minutes
Cooking time: 40 minutes
Servings: 4

Ingredients:
- 1 turkey breast, boneless, skinless and cubed
- ½ pound white mushrooms, halved
- 1/3 cup coconut aminos
- 2 garlic cloves, minced
- 2 tablespoons olive oil
- A pinch of black pepper
- 2 green onion, chopped
- 3 tablespoons garlic sauce
- 1 tablespoon rosemary, chopped

Directions:
1. Heat up a pan with the oil over medium heat, add the green onions, garlic sauce and the garlic and sauté for 5 minutes.
2. Add the meat and brown it for 5 minutes more.
3. Add the rest of the ingredients, introduce in the oven and bake at 390 degrees F for 30 minutes.
4. Divide the mix between plates and serve.

Nutrition: calories 154, fat 8.1, fiber 1.5, carbs 11.5, protein 9.8

Chicken and Olives Pan

Preparation time: 10 minutes
Cooking time: 25 minutes
Servings: 4

Ingredients:
- 1 pound chicken breasts, skinless, boneless and roughly cubed
- A pinch of black pepper
- 1 tablespoon avocado oil
- 1 red onion, chopped
- 1 cup coconut milk
- 1 tablespoon lemon juice
- 1 cup kalamata olives, pitted and sliced
- ¼ cup cilantro, chopped

Directions:
1. Heat up a pan with the oil over medium-high heat, add the onion and the meat and brown for 5 minutes.
2. Add the rest of the ingredients, toss, bring to a simmer and cook over medium heat for 20 minutes more.
3. Divide between plates and serve.

Nutrition: calories 409, fat 26.8, fiber 3.2, carbs 8.3, protein 34.9

Balsamic Turkey and Peach Mix

Preparation time: 10 minutes
Cooking time: 25 minutes
Servings: 4

Ingredients:
- 1 tablespoon avocado oil
- 1 turkey breast, skinless, boneless and sliced
- A pinch of black pepper
- 1 yellow onion, chopped
- 4 peaches, stones removed and cut into wedges
- ¼ cup balsamic vinegar
- 2 tablespoons chives, chopped

Directions:
1. Heat up a pan with the oil over medium-high heat, add the meat and the onion, toss and brown for 5 minutes.
2. Add the rest of the ingredients except the chives, toss gently and bake at 390 degrees F for 20 minutes.
3. Divide everything between plates and serve with the chives sprinkled on top.

Nutrition: calories 123, fat 1.6, fiber 3.3, carbs 18.8, protein 9.1

Coconut Chicken and Spinach

Preparation time: 10 minutes
Cooking time: 25 minutes
Servings: 4

Ingredients:
- 1 tablespoon avocado oil
- 1 pound chicken breast, skinless, boneless and cubed
- ½ teaspoon basil, dried
- A pinch of black pepper
- ¼ cup low-sodium veggie stock
- 2 cups baby spinach
- 2 shallots, chopped
- 2 garlic cloves, minced
- ½ teaspoon sweet paprika
- 2/3 cup coconut cream
- 2 tablespoons cilantro, chopped

Directions:
1. Heat up a pan with the oil over medium-high heat, add the meat, basil, black pepper and brown for 5 minutes.
2. Add the shallots and the garlic and cook for another 5 minutes.
3. Add the rest of the ingredients, toss, bring to a simmer and cook over medium heat fro 15 minutes more.
4. Divide between plates and serve hot.

Nutrition: calories 237, fat 12.9, fiber 1.6, carbs 4.7, protein 25.8

Chicken and Asparagus Mix

Preparation time: 10 minutes
Cooking time: 25 minutes
Servings: 4

Ingredients:
- 2 chicken breasts, skinless, boneless and cubed
- 2 tablespoons avocado oil
- 2 spring onions, chopped
- 1 bunch asparagus, trimmed and halved
- ½ teaspoon sweet paprika
- A pinch of black pepper
- 14 ounces canned tomatoes, no-salt-added, drained and chopped

Directions:
1. Heat up a pan with the oil over medium-high heat, add the meat and the spring onions, stir and cook for 5 minutes.
2. Add the asparagus and the other ingredients, toss, cover the pan and cook over medium heat for 20 minutes.
3. Divide everything between plates and serve.

Nutrition: calories 171, fat 6.4, fiber 2,6, carbs 6.4, protein 22.2

Turkey and Creamy Broccoli

Preparation time: 10 minutes
Cooking time: 25 minutes
Servings: 4

Ingredients:
- 1 tablespoon olive oil
- 1 big turkey breast, skinless, boneless and cubed
- 2 cups broccoli florets
- 2 shallots, chopped
- 2 garlic cloves, minced
- 1 tablespoon basil, chopped
- 1 tablespoon cilantro, chopped
- ½ cup coconut cream

Directions:
1. Heat up a pan with the oil over medium-high heat, add the meat, shallots and the garlic, toss and brown for 5 minutes.
2. Add the broccoli and the other ingredients, toss everything, cook for 20 minutes over medium heat, divide between plates and serve.

Nutrition: calories 165, fat 11.5, fiber 2.1, carbs 7.9, protein 9.6

Chicken and Dill Green Beans Mix

Preparation time: 10 minutes
Cooking time: 25 minutes
Servings: 4

Ingredients:
- 2 tablespoons olive oil
- 10 ounces green beans, trimmed and halved
- 1 yellow onion, chopped
- 1 tablespoon dill, chopped
- 2 chicken breasts, skinless, boneless and halved
- 2 cups tomato sauce, no-salt-added
- ½ teaspoon red pepper flakes, crushed

Directions:
1. Heat up a pan with the oil over medium-high heat, add the onion and the meat and brown it for 2 minutes on each side.
2. Add the green beans and the other ingredients, toss, introduce in the oven and bake at 380 degrees F fro 20 minutes.
3. Divide between plates and serve right away.

Nutrition: calories 391, fat 17.8, fiber 5, carbs 14.8, protein 43.9

Chicken and Chili Zucchini

Preparation time: 5 minutes
Cooking time: 25 minutes
Servings: 4

Ingredients:
- 1 pound chicken breasts, skinless, boneless and cubed
- 1 cup low-sodium chicken stock
- 2 zucchinis, roughly cubed
- 1 tablespoon olive oil
- 1 cup canned tomatoes, no-salt-added, chopped
- 1 yellow onion, chopped
- 1 teaspoon chili powder
- 1 tablespoon cilantro, chopped

Directions:
1. Heat up a pan with the oil over medium-high heat, add the meat and the onion, toss and brown for 5 minutes.
2. Add the zucchinis and the rest of the ingredients, toss gently, reduce the heat to medium and cook for 20 minutes.
3. Divide everything between plates and serve.

Nutrition: calories 284, fat 12.3, fiber 2.4, carbs 8, protein 35

Avocado and Chicken Mix

Preparation time: 10 minutes
Cooking time: 20 minutes
Servings: 4

Ingredients:
- 2 chicken breasts, skinless, boneless and halved
- Juice of ½ lemon
- 2 tablespoons olive oil
- 2 garlic cloves, minced
- ½ cup low-sodium veggie stock
- 1 avocado, peeled, pitted and cut into wedges
- A pinch of black pepper

Directions:
1. Heat up a pan with the oil over medium heat, add the garlic and the meat and brown for 2 minutes on each side.
2. Add the lemon juice and the other ingredients, bring to a simmer and cook over medium heat fro 15 minutes.
3. Divide the whole mix between plates and serve.

Nutrition: calories 436, fat 27.3, fiber 3.6, carbs 5.6, protein 41.8

Turkey and Bok Choy

Preparation time: 10 minutes
Cooking time: 20 minutes
Servings: 4

Ingredients:
- 1 turkey breast, boneless, skinless and roughly cubed
- 2 scallions, chopped
- 1 pound bok choy, torn
- 2 tablespoons olive oil
- ½ teaspoon ginger, grated
- A pinch of black pepper
- ½ cup low-sodium veggie stock

Directions:
1. Heat up a pot with the oil over medium-high heat, add the scallions and the ginger and sauté for 2 minutes.
2. Add the meat and brown for 5 minutes more.
3. Add the rest of the ingredients, toss, simmer for 13 minutes more, divide between plates and serve.

Nutrition: calories 125, fat 8, fiber 1.7, carbs 5.5, protein 9.3

Chicken with Red Onion Mix

Preparation time: 10 minutes
Cooking time: 25 minutes
Servings: 4

Ingredients:
- 2 chicken breasts, skinless, boneless and roughly cubed
- 3 red onions, sliced
- 2 tablespoons olive oil
- 1 cup low-sodium veggie stock
- A pinch of black pepper
- 1 tablespoon cilantro, chopped
- 1 tablespoon chives, chopped

Directions:
1. Heat up a pan with the oil over medium heat, add the onions and a pinch of black pepper, and sauté for 10 minutes stirring often.
2. Add the chicken and cook for 3 minutes more.
3. Add the rest of the ingredients, bring to a simmer and cook over medium heat for 12 minutes more.
4. Divide the chicken and onions mix between plates and serve.

Nutrition: calories 364, fat 17.5, fiber 2.1, carbs 8.8, protein 41.7

Hot Turkey and Rice

Preparation time: 10 minutes
Cooking time: 42 minutes
Servings: 4

Ingredients:
- 1 turkey breast, skinless, boneless and cubed
- 1 cup white rice
- 2 cups low-sodium veggie stock
- 1 teaspoon hot paprika
- 2 small Serrano peppers, chopped
- 2 garlic cloves, minced
- 2 tablespoons olive oil
- ½ red bell pepper chopped
- A pinch of black pepper

Directions:
1. Heat up a pan with the oil over medium heat, add the Serrano peppers and garlic and sauté for 2 minutes.
2. Add the meat and brown it for 5 minutes.
3. Add the rice and the other ingredients, bring to a simmer and cook over medium heat for 35 minutes.
4. Stir, divide between plates and serve.

Nutrition: calories 271, fat 7.7, fiber 1.7, carbs 42, protein 7.8

Lemony Leek and Chicken

Preparation time: 10 minutes
Cooking time: 40 minutes
Servings: 4

Ingredients:
- 1 pound chicken breast, skinless, boneless and cubed
- A pinch of black pepper
- 2 tablespoons avocado oil
- 1 tablespoon tomato sauce, no-salt-added
- 1 cup low-sodium veggie stock
- 4 leek, roughly chopped
- ½ cup lemon juice

Directions:
1. Heat up a pan with the oil over medium heat, add the leeks, toss and sauté for 10 minutes.
2. Add the chicken and the other ingredients, toss, cook over medium heat for 20 minutes more, divide between plates and serve.

Nutrition: calories 199, fat 13.3, fiber 5, carbs 7.6, protein 17.4

Turkey with Savoy Cabbage Mix

Preparation time: 10 minutes
Cooking time: 35 minutes
Servings: 4

Ingredients:
- 1 big turkey breast, skinless, boneless and cubed
- 1 cup low-sodium chicken stock
- 1 tablespoon coconut oil, melted
- 1 Savoy cabbage, shredded
- 1 teaspoon chili powder
- 1 teaspoon sweet paprika
- 1 garlic clove, minced
- 1 yellow onion, chopped
- A pinch of salt and black pepper

Directions:
1. Heat up a pan with the oil over medium heat, add the meat and brown for 5 minutes.
2. Add the garlic and the onion, toss and sauté for 5 minutes more.
3. Add the cabbage and the other ingredients, toss, bring to a simmer and cook over medium heat for 25 minutes.
4. Divide everything between plates and serve.

Nutrition: calories 299, fat 14.5, fiber 5, carbs 8.8, protein 12.6

Chicken with Paprika Scallions

Preparation time: 10 minutes
Cooking time: 30 minutes
Servings: 4

Ingredients:
- 1 pound chicken breast, skinless, boneless and sliced
- 4 scallions, chopped
- 1 tablespoon olive oil
- 1 tablespoon sweet paprika
- 1 cup low-sodium chicken stock
- 1 tablespoon ginger, grated
- 1 teaspoon oregano, dried
- 1 teaspoon cumin, ground
- 1 teaspoon allspice, ground
- ½ cup cilantro, chopped
- A pinch of black pepper

Directions:
1. Heat up a pan with the oil over medium heat, add the scallions and the meat and brown for 5 minutes.
2. Add the rest of the ingredients, toss, introduce in the oven and bake at 390 degrees F for 25 minutes.
3. Divide the chicken and scallions mix between plates and serve.

Nutrition: calories 295, fat 12.5, fiber 6.9, carbs 22.4, protein 15.6

Chicken and Mustard Sauce

Preparation time: 10 minutes
Cooking time: 35 minutes
Servings: 4

Ingredients:
- 1 pound chicken thighs, boneless and skinless
- 1 tablespoon avocado oil
- 2 tablespoons mustard
- 1 shallot, chopped
- 1 cup low-sodium chicken stock
- A pinch of salt and black pepper
- 3 garlic cloves, minced
- ½ teaspoon basil, dried

Directions:
1. Heat up a pan with the oil over medium heat, add the shallot, garlic and the chicken and brown everything for 5 minutes.
2. Add the mustard and the rest of the ingredients, toss gently, bring to a simmer and cook over medium heat for 30 minutes.
3. Divide everything between plates and serve hot.

Nutrition: calories 299, fat 15.5, fiber 6.6, carbs 30.3, protein 12.5

Chicken and Celery Mix

Preparation time: 10 minutes
Cooking time: 35 minutes
Servings: 4

Ingredients:
- A pinch of black pepper
- 2 pounds chicken breast, skinless, boneless and cubed
- 2 tablespoons olive oil
- 1 cup celery, chopped
- 3 garlic cloves, minced
- 1 poblano pepper, chopped
- 1 cup low-sodium veggie stock
- 1 teaspoon chili powder
- 2 tablespoons chives, chopped

Directions:
1. Heat up a pan with the oil over medium heat, add the garlic, celery and poblano pepper, toss and cook for 5 minutes.
2. Add the meat, toss and cook for another 5 minutes.
3. Add the rest of the ingredients except the chives, bring to a simmer and cook over medium heat for 25 minutes more.
4. Divide the whole mix between plates and serve with the chives sprinkled on top.

Nutrition: calories 305, fat 18, fiber 13.4, carbs 22.5, protein 6

Lime Turkey with Baby Potatoes

Preparation time: 10 minutes
Cooking time: 40 minutes
Servings: 4

Ingredients:
- 1 turkey breast, skinless, boneless and sliced
- 2 tablespoons olive oil
- 1 pound baby potatoes, peeled and halved
- 1 tablespoon sweet paprika
- 1 yellow onion, chopped
- 1 teaspoon chili powder
- 1 teaspoon rosemary, dried
- 2 cups low-sodium chicken stock
- A pinch of black pepper
- Zest of 1 lime, grated
- 1 tablespoon lime juice
- 1 tablespoon cilantro, chopped

Directions:
1. Heat up a pan with the oil over medium heat, add the onion, chili powder and the rosemary, toss and sauté for 5 minutes.
2. Add the meat, and brown for 5 minutes more.
3. Add the potatoes and the rest of the ingredients except the cilantro, toss gently, bring to a simmer and cook over medium heat for 30 minutes.
4. Divide the mix between plates and serve with the cilantro sprinkled on top.

Nutrition: calories 345, fat 22.2, fiber 12.3, carbs 34.5, protein 16.4

Chicken with Mustard Greens

Preparation time: 10 minutes
Cooking time: 25 minutes
Servings: 4

Ingredients:
- 2 chicken breasts, skinless, boneless and cubed
- 3 cups mustard greens
- 1 cup canned tomatoes, no-salt-added, chopped
- 1 red onion, chopped
- 2 tablespoons avocado oil
- 1 teaspoon oregano, dried
- 2 garlic cloves, minced
- 1 tablespoon chives, chopped
- 1 tablespoon balsamic vinegar
- A pinch of black pepper

Directions:
1. Heat up a pan with the oil over medium-high heat, add the onion and the garlic and sauté for 5 minutes.
2. Add the meat and brown it for 5 minutes more.
3. Add the greens, tomatoes and the other ingredients, toss, cook for 20 minutes over medium heat, divide between plates and serve.

Nutrition: calories 290, fat 12.3, fiber 6.7, carbs 22.30, protein 14.3

Baked Chicken and Apples

Preparation time: 10 minutes
Cooking time: 50 minutes
Servings: 4

Ingredients:
- 2 pounds chicken thighs, boneless and skinless
- 2 tablespoons olive oil
- 2 red onions, sliced
- A pinch of black pepper
- 1 teaspoon thyme, dried
- 1 teaspoon basil, dried
- 1 cup green apples, cored and roughly cubed
- 2 garlic cloves, minced
- 2 cups low-sodium chicken stock
- 1 tablespoon lemon juice
- 1 cup tomatoes, cubed
- 1 tablespoon cilantro, chopped

Directions:
1. Heat up a pan with the oil over medium-high heat, add the onions and garlic, and sauté for 5 minutes.
2. Add the chicken and brown for another 5 minutes.
3. Add the thyme, basil and the other ingredients, toss gently, introduce in the oven and bake at 390 degrees F for 40 minutes.
4. Divide the chicken and apples mix between plates and serve.

Nutrition: calories 290, fat 12.3, fiber 4, carbs 15.7, protein 10

Chipotle Chicken

Preparation time: 10 minutes
Cooking time: 1 hour
Servings: 6

Ingredients:
- 2 pounds chicken thighs, boneless and skinless
- 1 yellow onion, chopped
- 2 tablespoons olive oil
- 3 garlic cloves, minced
- 1 tablespoon coriander seeds, ground
- 1 teaspoon cumin, ground
- 1 cup low-sodium chicken stock
- 4 tablespoons chipotle chili paste
- A pinch of black pepper
- 1 tablespoon coriander, chopped

Directions:
1. Heat up a pan with the oil over medium heat, add the onion and the garlic and sauté for 5 minutes.
2. Add the meat and brown for 5 minutes more.
3. Add the rest of the ingredients, toss, introduce everything in the oven and bake at 390 degrees F for 50 minutes.
4. Divide the whole mix between plates and serve.

Nutrition: calories 280, fat 12.1, fiber 6.3, carbs 15.7, protein 12

Herbed Turkey

Preparation time: 10 minutes
Cooking time: 35 minutes
Servings: 4

Ingredients:
- 1 big turkey breast, boneless, skinless and sliced
- 1 tablespoon chives, chopped
- 1 tablespoon oregano, chopped
- 1 tablespoon basil, chopped
- 1 tablespoon coriander, chopped
- 2 shallots, chopped
- 2 tablespoons olive oil
- 1 cup low-sodium chicken stock
- 1 cup tomatoes, cubed
- Salt and black pepper to the taste

Directions:
1. Heat up a pan with the oil over medium heat, add the shallots and the meat and brown for 5 minutes.
2. Add the chives and the other ingredients, toss, bring to a simmer and cook over medium heat for 30 minutes.
3. Divide the mix between plates and serve.

Nutrition: calories 290, fat 11.9, fiber 5.5, carbs 16.2, protein 9

Chicken and Ginger Sauce

Preparation time: 10 minutes
Cooking time: 35 minutes
Servings: 4

Ingredients:
- 1 pound chicken breast, skinless, boneless and cubed
- 1 tablespoon ginger, grated
- 1 tablespoon olive oil
- 2 shallots, chopped
- 1 tablespoon balsamic vinegar
- A pinch of black pepper
- ¾ cup low-sodium chicken stock
- 1 tablespoon basil, chopped

Directions:
1. Heat up a pan with the oil over medium heat, add the shallots and the ginger, stir and sauté for 5 minutes.
2. Add the rest of the ingredients except the chicken, toss, bring to a simmer and cook for 5 minutes more.
3. Add the chicken, toss, simmer the whole mix for 25 minutes, divide between plates and serve.

Nutrition: calories 294, fat 15.5, fiber 3, carbs 15.4, protein 13.1

Chicken and Corn

Preparation time: 10 minutes
Cooking time: 35 minutes
Servings: 4

Ingredients:
- 2 pounds chicken breast, skinless, boneless and halved
- 2 cups corn
- 2 tablespoons avocado oil
- A pinch of black pepper
- 1 teaspoon smoked paprika
- 1 bunch green onions, chopped
- 1 cup low-sodium chicken stock

Directions:
1. Heat up a pan with the oil over medium-high heat, add the green onions, stir and sauté them for 5 minutes.
2. Add the chicken and brown it for 5 minutes more.
3. Add the corn and the other ingredients, toss, introduce the pan in the oven and cook at 390 degrees F for 25 minutes.
4. Divide the mix between plates and serve.

Nutrition: calories 270, fat 12.4, fiber 5.2, carbs 12, protein 9

Curry Turkey and Quinoa

Preparation time: 10 minutes
Cooking time: 40 minutes
Servings: 4

Ingredients:
- 1 pound turkey breast, skinless, boneless and cubed
- 1 tablespoon olive oil
- 1 cup quinoa
- 2 cups low-sodium chicken stock
- 1 tablespoon lime juice
- 1 tablespoon parsley, chopped
- A pinch of black pepper
- 1 tablespoon red curry paste

Directions:
1. Heat up a pan with the oil over medium-high heat, add the meat and brown it for 5 minutes.
2. Add the quinoa and the rest of the ingredients, toss, bring to a simmer and cook over medium heat for 35 minutes.
3. Divide everything between plates and serve.

Nutrition: calories 310, fat 8.5, fiber 11, carbs 30.4, protein 16.3

Turkey and Cumin Parsnips

Preparation time: 10 minutes
Cooking time: 40 minutes
Servings: 4

Ingredients:
- 1 pound turkey breast, skinless, boneless and cubed
- 2 parsnips, peeled and cubed
- 2 teaspoons cumin, ground
- 1 tablespoon parsley, chopped
- 2 tablespoons avocado oil
- 2 shallots, chopped
- 1 cup low-sodium chicken stock
- 4 garlic cloves, minced
- A pinch of black pepper

Directions:
1. Heat up a pan with the oil over medium heat, add the shallots and the garlic and sauté for 5 minutes.
2. Add the turkey, toss and cook for 5 minutes more.
3. Add the parsnips and the other ingredients, toss, simmer over medium heat for 30 minutes more, divide between plates and serve.

Nutrition: calories 284, fat 18.2, fiber 4, carbs 16.7, protein 12.3

Turkey and Cilantro Chickpeas

Preparation time: 10 minutes
Cooking time: 40 minutes
Servings: 4

Ingredients:
- 1 cup canned chickpeas, no-salt-added, drained
- 1 cup low-sodium chicken stock
- 1 pound turkey breast, skinless, boneless and cubed
- A pinch of black pepper
- 1 teaspoon oregano, dried
- 1 teaspoon nutmeg, ground
- 2 tablespoons olive oil
- 1 yellow onion, chopped
- 1 green bell pepper, chopped
- 1 cup cilantro, chopped

Directions:
1. Heat up a pan with the oil over medium heat, add the onion, bell pepper and the meat and cook for 10 minutes stirring often.
2. Add the rest of the ingredients, toss, bring to a simmer and cook over medium heat for 30 minutes.
3. Divide the mix between plates and serve.

Nutrition: calories 304, fat 11.2, fiber 4.5, carbs 22.2, protein 17

Turkey and Curry Lentils

Preparation time: 10 minutes
Cooking time: 40 minutes
Servings: 4

Ingredients:
- 2 pounds turkey breast, skinless, boneless and cubed
- 1 cup canned lentils, no-salt-added, drained and rinsed
- 1 tablespoon green curry paste
- 1 teaspoon garam masala
- 2 tablespoons olive oil
- 1 yellow onion, chopped
- 1 garlic clove, minced
- A pinch of black pepper
- 1 tablespoon cilantro, chopped

Directions:
1. Heat up a pan with the oil over medium heat, add the onion, garlic and the meat and brown for 5 minutes stirring often.
2. Add the lentils and the other ingredients, bring to a simmer and cook over medium heat for 35 minutes.
3. Divide the mix between plates and serve.

Nutrition: calories 489, fat 12.1, fiber 16.4, carbs 42.4, protein 51.5

Turkey with Beans and Olives

Preparation time: 10 minutes
Cooking time: 35 minutes
Servings: 4

Ingredients:
- 1 cup black beans, no-salt-added and drained
- 1 cup green olives, pitted and halved
- 1 pound turkey breast, skinless, boneless and sliced
- 1 tablespoon cilantro, chopped
- 1 cup tomato sauce, no-salt-added
- 1 tablespoon olive oil

Directions:
1. Grease a baking dish with the oil, arrange the turkey slices inside, add the other ingredients as well, introduce in the oven and bake at 380 degrees F for 35 minutes.
2. Divide between plates and serve.

Nutrition: calories 331, fat 6.4, fiber 9, carbs 38.5, protein 30.7

Chicken and Tomato Quinoa

Preparation time: 10 minutes
Cooking time: 35 minutes
Servings: 8

Ingredients:
- 1 tablespoon olive oil
- 2 pounds chicken breasts, skinless, boneless and halved
- 1 teaspoon rosemary, ground
- A pinch of salt and black pepper
- 2 shallots, chopped
- 1 tablespoon olive oil
- 3 tablespoons low-sodium tomato sauce
- 2 cups quinoa, already cooked

Directions:
1. Heat up a pan with the oil over medium-high heat, add the meat and shallots and brown for 2 minutes on each side.
2. Add the rosemary and the other ingredients, toss, introduce in the oven and cook at 370 degrees F for 30 minutes.
3. Divide the mix between plates and serve.

Nutrition: calories 406, fat 14.5, fiber 3.1, carbs 28.1, protein 39

Allspice Chicken Wings

Preparation time: 10 minutes
Cooking time: 20 minutes
Servings: 4

Ingredients:
- 2 pounds chicken wings
- 2 teaspoons allspice, ground
- 2 tablespoons avocado oil
- 5 garlic cloves, minced
- Black pepper to the taste
- 2 tablespoons chives, chopped

Directions:
1. In a bowl, combine the chicken wings with the allspice and the other ingredients and toss well.
2. Arrange the chicken wings in a roasting pan and bake at 400 degrees F for 20 minutes.
3. Divide the chicken wings between plates and serve.

Nutrition: calories 449, fat 17.8, fiber 0.6, carbs 2.4, protein 66.1

Chicken and Snow Peas

Preparation time: 10 minutes
Cooking time: 30 minutes
Servings: 4

Ingredients:
- 2 pounds chicken breasts, skinless, boneless and cubed
- 2 cups snow peas
- 2 tablespoons olive oil
- 1 red onion, chopped
- 1 cup canned tomato sauce, no-salt-added
- 2 tablespoons parsley, chopped
- A pinch of black pepper

Directions:
1. Heat up a pan with the oil over medium heat, add the onion and the meat and brown for 5 minutes.
2. Add the peas and the rest of the ingredients, bring to a simmer and cook over medium heat for 25 minutes.
3. Divide the mix between plates and serve.

Nutrition: calories 551, fat 24.2, fiber 3.8, carbs 11.7, protein 69.4